plant-based diet for a complete beginner

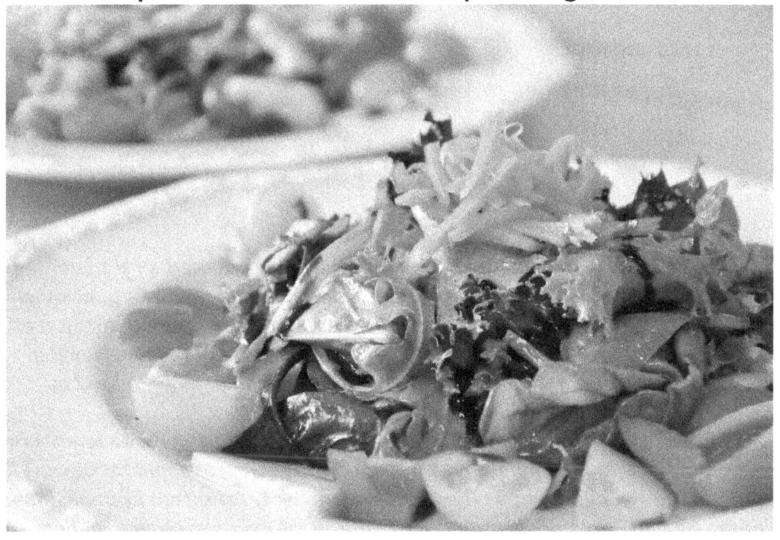

Very easy and healthy budget meal prep

SANTA G HOOPER

Table of content

INTRODUCTION

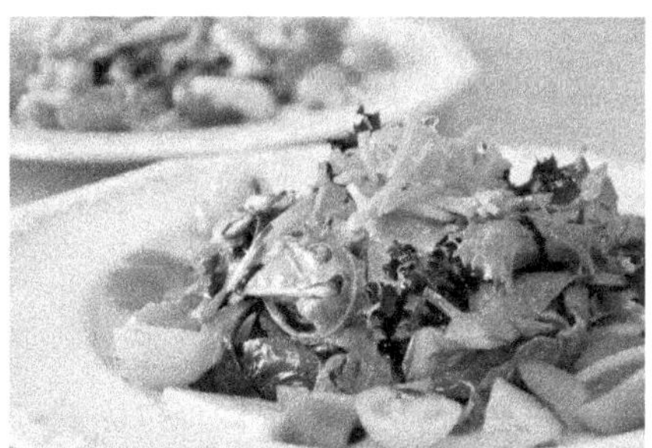

Embarking on a plant-based diet is a powerful choice for your health, the planet, and your wallet. But making this shift need not be daunting or expensive. Welcome to "Plant-Based Diet: Easy and Healthy Budget Meal Prep," your comprehensive guide to unlocking the full potential of affordable, plant-powered eating.

In this journey, we will demystify the world of plant-based nutrition and meal prep, proving that vibrant, wholesome meals can be accessible to everyone. Whether you're a student on a tight budget, a busy professional seeking convenient options, or simply someone looking to improve their health without breaking the bank, this guide has you covered.

We'll explore the art of smart grocery shopping, discovering wallet-friendly alternatives to traditional ingredients, and mastering the art of batch cooking. With an array of delicious, nutrient-rich recipes designed for simplicity and cost-effectiveness, you'll soon realize that a plant-based diet is not only good for your health but also your savings account.

Get ready to embrace a lifestyle that benefits your well-being, the environment, and your finances. Let's embark on this journey together, creating a world where easy, healthy, and budget-friendly plant-based meals are the norm.

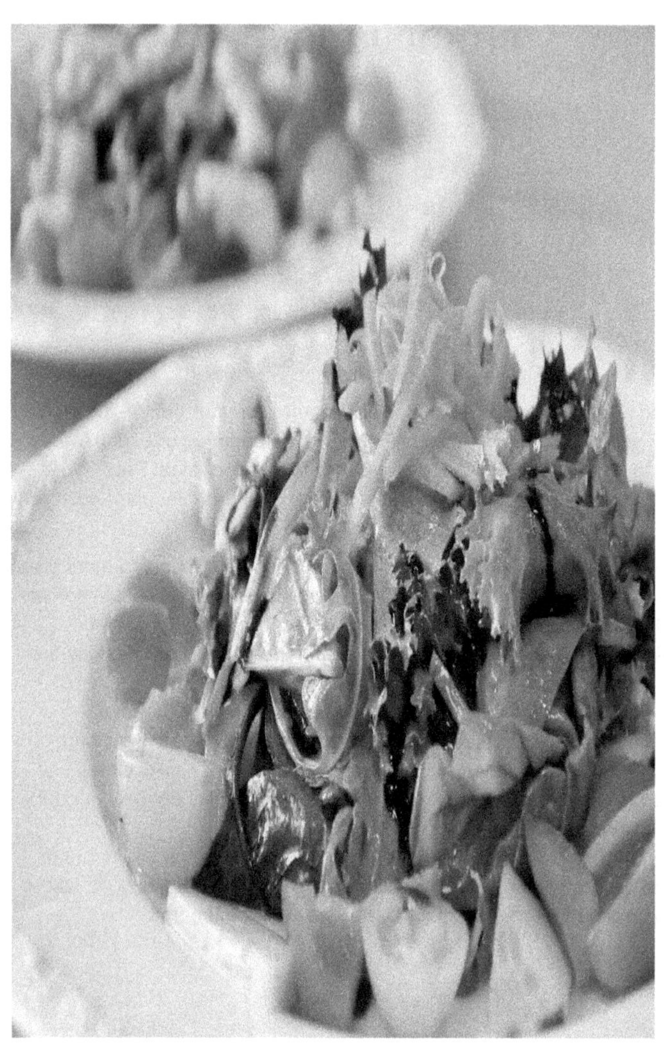

CHAPTER ONE

Meaning of a Plant-Based Diet

A plant-based diet is a dietary approach centered on the consumption of foods derived primarily from plant sources, including fruits, vegetables, whole grains, legumes, nuts, seeds, and plant-based proteins. It excludes or significantly limits the intake of animal products such as meat, dairy, and eggs. A plant-based diet emphasizes whole, minimally processed foods and places a strong focus on the health and environmental benefits associated with reduced animal product consumption."

This definition provides an overview of what a plant-based diet entails and its key principles.

Benefits of a plant-based diet

Bettered Heart Health Plant- grounded diets are associated with a lower threat of heart complaint. They tend to be lower in saturated fat and cholesterol, which can reduce the risk of high blood pressure and clogged arteries.

Weight Management: Plant-based diets are often naturally lower in calories and higher in fiber, which can help with weight management and weight loss goals.

Lower Risk of Chronic Diseases: Research suggests that plant-based diets may reduce the risk of chronic diseases such as type 2 diabetes, certain types of cancer, and hypertension.

Better Digestive Health: A diet rich in fiber from plant foods can promote healthy digestion and reduce the risk of constipation and other digestive issues.

Reduced Environmental Impact: Plant-based diets have a lower carbon footprint and contribute to reduced greenhouse gas emissions, making them more environmentally sustainable.

Ethical Considerations: Many people choose plant-based diets for ethical reasons, as they avoid the harm and suffering associated with the production of animal products.

Improved Gut Health: Plant-based diets can promote a diverse and healthy gut microbiome, which is linked to overall well-being.

Anti-Inflammatory Properties: Some plant-based foods, like berries, leafy greens, and nuts, are rich in anti-inflammatory compounds that can help reduce inflammation in the body.

Enhanced Longevity: Studies suggest that plant-based diets may be associated with a longer lifespan and a lower risk of premature death.
Weight Loss and Management: Many people find it easier to maintain a healthy weight or lose excess weight on a plant-based diet due to its lower calorie density and higher fiber content.
It's important to note that the specific benefits can vary from person to person, and individual dietary choices within a plant-based framework can influence outcomes. Additionally, a well-balanced and nutrient-rich plant-based diet is key to maximizing these benefits. Consulting with a healthcare provider or registered dietitian can provide personalized guidance for adopting a plant-based diet that meets your health goals.

CHAPTER TWO

TYPES OF PLANT-BASED DIET

VEGAN DIET   A vegan diet is a dietary and lifestyle choice that excludes all animal products and by-products. It is a form of vegetarianism but goes a step further by eliminating not only meat but also all animal-derived foods, including dairy, eggs, and honey. A vegan diet is entirely plant-based.

Here are some key aspects of a vegan diet

Plant Foods: A vegan diet is based on plant foods such as fruits, vegetables, whole grains, legumes (beans, lentils, chickpeas), nuts, seeds, and plant-based protein sources like tofu and tempeh.

Exclusion of Animal Products: Vegans do not consume any animal products, including red meat, poultry, seafood, dairy products (milk, cheese, yogurt), eggs, and honey.

Emphasis on Whole Foods: Many vegans emphasize whole, minimally processed foods to ensure a balanced and nutritious diet. This includes avoiding highly processed vegan substitutes like vegan burgers and vegan hot dogs.

Health Benefits: A vegan diet is associated with several health benefits, including a reduced risk of heart disease, lower blood pressure, improved weight management, and a decreased risk of certain types of cancer. It's often chosen for its potential health advantages.

Ethical and Environmental Considerations: Many vegans choose this lifestyle for ethical reasons, as they believe it reduces harm to animals and promotes animal welfare. Additionally, a vegan diet is seen as a more sustainable choice with a lower environmental impact due to reduced greenhouse gas emissions associated with animal agriculture.

Variety of Vegan Foods: A vegan diet is not limited to salads and vegetables. It includes a wide variety of foods, and there are vegan alternatives for many traditional animal-based products, including plant-based milk, cheese, ice cream, and meat substitutes.

Supplementation: Some vegans may need to supplement certain nutrients such as vitamin B12, vitamin D, and omega-3 fatty acids since they are less readily available in a strict plant-based diet.

It's important to note that the specific benefits can vary from person to person, and individual dietary choices within a plant-based framework can influence outcomes. Additionally, a well-balanced and nutrient-rich plant-based diet is key to maximizing these benefits. Consulting with a healthcare provider or registered dietitian can provide personalized guidance for adopting a plant-based diet that meets your health goals.

VEGETARIAN DIET

A vegetarian diet is a dietary pattern that excludes the consumption of meat and seafood but allows for the consumption of other animal-derived products, such as dairy, eggs, and honey. There are different variations of vegetarian diets, each with its level of animal product exclusion. Here are some common types:

Lacto-Ovo Vegetarian: Lacto-ovo vegetarians are individuals who follow a vegetarian diet that excludes meat, poultry, and seafood but include dairy products (Lacto) and eggs (Ovo) in their diet. They abstain from consuming animal flesh but still incorporate animal-derived products like milk, cheese, yogurt, and eggs into their meals. This dietary choice allows them to obtain essential nutrients like protein, calcium, and vitamin B12 from dairy and egg sources while avoiding meat.

Lacto-Vegetarian: Lacto-vegetarians exclude meat, seafood, and eggs but include dairy products in their diet.

Ovo-Vegetarian: Ovo-vegetarians exclude meat, seafood, and dairy products but include eggs in their diet.

Pescatarian: Pescatarians rule out meat but include seafood in their diet. They may or may not eat dairy and eggs.

Flexitarian or Semi-Vegetarian: Flexitarians primarily follow a vegetarian diet but occasionally include small amounts of meat or seafood in their meals.

Key points about a vegetarian diet *Plant-Based Focus:* A vegetarian diet places a strong emphasis on plant foods, including fruits, vegetables, whole grains, legumes, nuts, and seeds.

Health Benefits: Research suggests that vegetarian diets may offer various health benefits, such as a reduced risk of heart disease, lower blood pressure, better weight management, and improved longevity.

Ethical and Environmental Considerations: Many people choose a vegetarian diet for ethical reasons, as it reduces harm to animals, and for environmental reasons, as it is often viewed as a more sustainable choice compared to omnivorous diets.

Variety of Vegetarian Foods: There is a wide variety of delicious vegetarian foods available, and vegetarian diets can be nutritionally complete when well-balanced. Vegetarian alternatives to animal products, such as plant-based milk, cheese, and meat substitutes, are widely available.

Potential Nutrient Considerations: While a vegetarian diet can be nutritious, individuals need to pay attention to obtaining essential nutrients like protein, iron, calcium, vitamin B12, and omega-3 fatty acids. These nutrients may require special attention or supplementation in some cases.

It's important to note that vegetarian diets can vary in their nutritional quality and composition, depending on individual food choices. Consulting with a registered dietitian or healthcare provider can help ensure that a vegetarian diet meets all nutritional needs and preferences.

FLEXITARIAN DIET.

A flexitarian diet, often referred to as a semi-vegetarian or flexible vegetarian diet, is a dietary pattern that is primarily plant-based but allows for occasional consumption of meat or other animal products. Flexitarians primarily focus on plant-based foods while incorporating small amounts of animal-derived foods into their diet on occasion. Here are some key features of a flexitarian diet:

Plant-Based Emphasis: Flexitarians prioritize plant foods, including fruits, vegetables, whole grains, legumes (beans, lentils, chickpeas), nuts, seeds, and plant-based protein sources like tofu and tempeh.

Occasional Meat Consumption: Flexitarians may include small portions of meat, poultry, or seafood in their meals, but these are not central components of their diet. The frequency and quantity of animal products consumed can vary widely among individuals following a flexitarian approach.

Health Benefits: The flexitarian diet is associated with potential health benefits similar to those of vegetarian diets, including reduced risk of heart disease, lower blood pressure, improved weight management, and enhanced overall well-being.

Flexibility: The flexibility of the flexitarian diet allows individuals to adapt their food choices to their preferences, health goals, and ethical considerations. Some flexitarians may choose to eat meat only occasionally, while others may include it more regularly.

Ethical and Environmental Considerations: Many people choose a flexitarian diet for ethical and environmental reasons. By reducing their meat consumption, flexitarians aim to reduce the environmental impact of their diet and minimize harm to animals.

Nutrient Considerations: Flexitarians need to pay attention to obtaining essential nutrients like protein, iron, calcium, vitamin B12, and omega-3 fatty acids, especially if they limit animal products. Careful meal planning can help ensure that nutritional needs are met.

Variety of Foods: A flexitarian diet allows for a wide variety of foods and culinary options, incorporating both plant-based and occasional animal-based dishes.

Sustainability: The flexitarian diet aligns with sustainability goals by reducing the overall demand for meat production, which can have a significant environmental impact.

Overall, a flexitarian diet provides individuals with the flexibility to enjoy the health benefits and ethical considerations of a plant-based diet while occasionally incorporating animal products to suit their preferences and nutritional needs. It is a balanced and adaptable approach to eating that can be tailored to individual lifestyles and values.

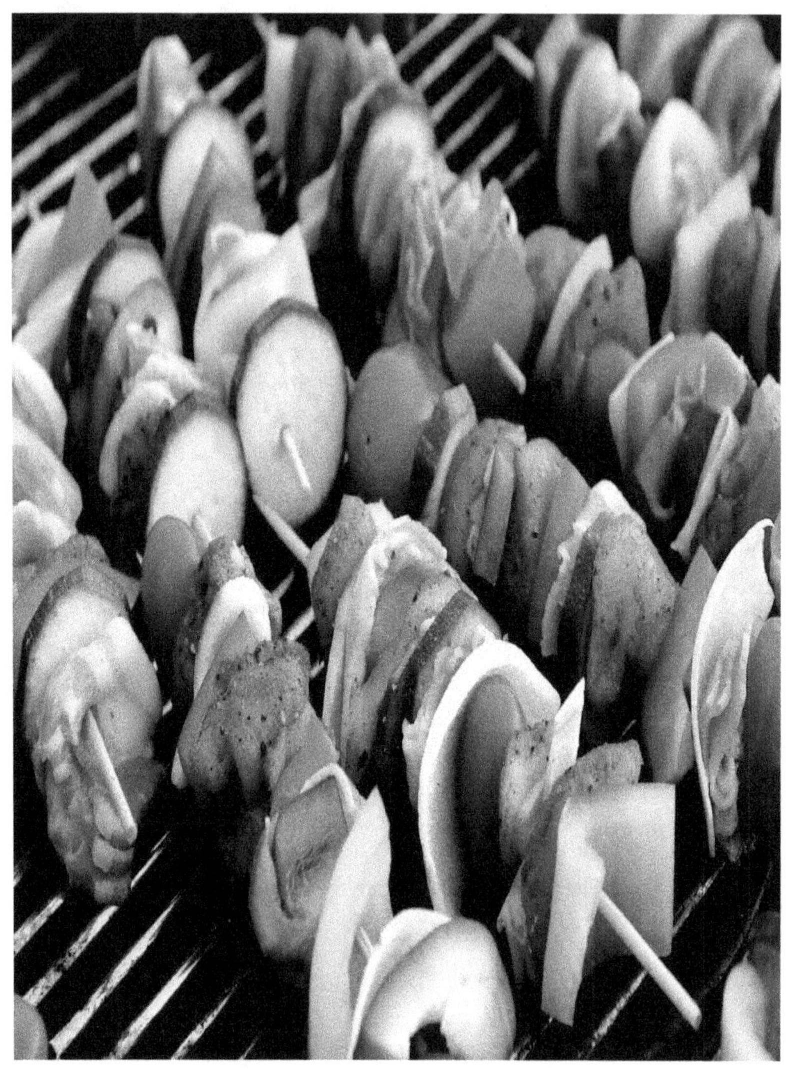

CHAPTER THREE

TRANSITIONING TO A PLANT-BASED DIET

Tips for Beginners

Transitioning to a plant-based diet can be both exciting and rewarding, but it may also come with challenges, especially for beginners. Here are some tips to help you get started on a plant-based journey:

1. Instruct yourself to grasp the time to master plant-based nutrition. Understand the nutrients you need, where to find them in plant foods, and how to create balanced meals.

2. Start Gradually: If going completely vegan seems daunting, consider easing into it. Begin by designating a few days each week as plant-based and gradually increase the number of meatless days.

3. Explore New Foods: Embrace the opportunity to discover new fruits, vegetables, grains, and legumes. trial with distinctive methods and cuisines to keep your tables innovative.

4. Plan Your Meals: Meal planning is essential. Make a weekly meal plan, create a shopping list, and prep ingredients in advance to make plant-based cooking more convenient.

5. Stock Up on Staples: Keep plant-based pantry staples on hand, such as whole grains, beans, lentils, canned tomatoes, herbs, and spices. These items can serve as the foundation for many meals.

6. Find Vegan Substitutes: There are vegan alternatives for most animal-based products, including plant-based milk, cheese, and meat substitutes. Experiment with these options to ease the transition.

7. Read Labels: Be vigilant about reading food labels, as some processed foods may contain hidden animal-derived ingredients. Look for vegan certifications when available.

8. Learn to Cook: Cooking your meals gives you control over what you eat and allows you to create flavorful and satisfying plant-based dishes. Invest in some basic cooking skills if you're not already a seasoned cook.

9. Balance Your Nutrients: Pay attention to getting a variety of nutrients, including protein, iron, calcium, vitamin B12, and omega-3 fatty acids. Consider consulting a dietitian for substantiated advice.

10. Stay Doused Drink plenitude of water throughout the day to stay doused. Herbal teas and infused water can add flavor without extra calories.

11. Embrace Whole Foods: Focus on whole, unprocessed foods like fruits, vegetables, whole grains, nuts, and seeds. Minimize your intake of highly processed vegan alternatives.

12. Join a Community: Connect with others on a plant-based journey through social media, online forums, or local vegan or vegetarian groups. Sharing experiences and recipes can be motivating and informative.

13. Be Patient: Be kind to yourself during the transition. It's okay to have occasional slip-ups or cravings for non-plant-based foods. Progress, not perfection, is key.

14. Try Meatless Mondays: Start with a simple goal, like participating in Meatless Mondays, and gradually expand from there.

15. Explore Restaurants: Many restaurants now offer vegan options. Explore vegan-friendly eateries in your area or check menus in advance when dining out.

Remember that transitioning to a plant-based diet is a personal journey, and there is no one-size-fits-all approach. Listen to your body, make adjustments as needed, and enjoy the process of discovering delicious and nutritious plant-based foods.

Overcoming Challenges   Transitioning to a plant-based diet can come with its challenges, but with determination and some strategies, you can overcome them.

Currently are some common challenges and tips for overmastering them

1. Lack of Variety: Challenge: You might feel like you're eating the same foods over and over.

Tip: Explore new recipes and cuisines. Try one new plant-based food item or recipe each week to keep your meals exciting and diverse.

2. Social Pressure: Challenge: Social gatherings and dining out with non-vegan friends and family can be challenging.

Tip: Communicate your dietary choices with your loved ones. Offer to bring a vegan dish to share at gatherings, or choose restaurants with vegan-friendly options.

3. Nutrient Concerns: Challenge: Worries about getting enough protein, iron, calcium, or other nutrients.

Tip: Plan balanced meals that include a variety of plant-based protein sources, and leafy greens for iron and calcium, and consider supplements if needed.

4. Cravings: Challenge: Cravings for non-vegan comfort foods.

Tip: Find plant-based alternatives or vegan versions of your favorite comfort foods. Cravings often diminish over time as your taste buds adjust.

5. Label Reading: Challenge: Identifying hidden animal-derived ingredients in processed foods.

Tip: Learn to read labels carefully, and look for vegan certifications or symbols. Many apps and websites can help you identify vegan products.

6. Dining Out: Challenge: Limited vegan options at restaurants.

Tip: Research vegan-friendly restaurants in your area before dining out. Be polite but assertive when asking for vegan modifications to menu items.

7. Time and Convenience: Challenge: The perception that plant-based cooking takes more time and effort.

Tip: Plan meals, batch cook, and use time-saving kitchen gadgets. Many plant-based meals can be quick and simple to prepare.

8. Support: Challenge: Feeling isolated or unsupported in your plant-based journey.

Tip: Connect with the plant-based community online or in person. Share your experiences, ask questions, and seek advice and support from like-minded individuals.

9. Food Costs: Challenge: Concerns about the cost of specialty vegan products.

Tip: Focus on budget-friendly plant-based staples like beans, lentils, rice, oats, and seasonal fruits and vegetables. Buy in bulk when possible.

10. Patience: Challenge: Expecting instant results or perfection.

Tip: Be patient with yourself and recognize that transitioning takes time. Small steps and gradual changes are often more sustainable.

Remember that challenges are a normal part of any significant lifestyle change. Stay committed to your plant-based goals, keep learning, and be flexible in finding solutions that work for you. With time and experience, the challenges will become easier to overcome, and you'll reap the many benefits of a plant-based lifestyle.

Storage and Reheating of plant-based foods and vegetables

Certainly! Storage and reheating of food are important aspects of food safety and convenience. Here are some general guidelines:

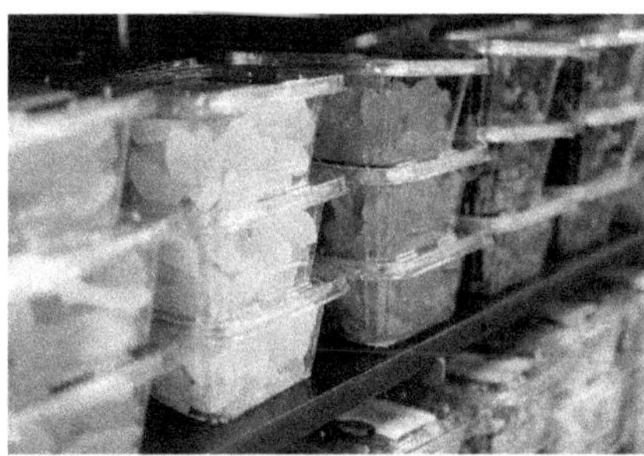

Perishable foods like meats, dairy, and leftovers should be stored in the refrigerator at temperatures below 40°F (4°C) to slow down bacterial growth.

Freezing: You can freeze many foods to extend their shelf life. Make sure to use watertight holders or freezer bags to help the freezer burn.

Labeling: Label containers with the date of storage to track freshness and ensure you use them within a reasonable time.

Food Safety: Follow the "first in, first out" (FIFO) principle, using older items before newer ones to prevent food waste.

Reheating:

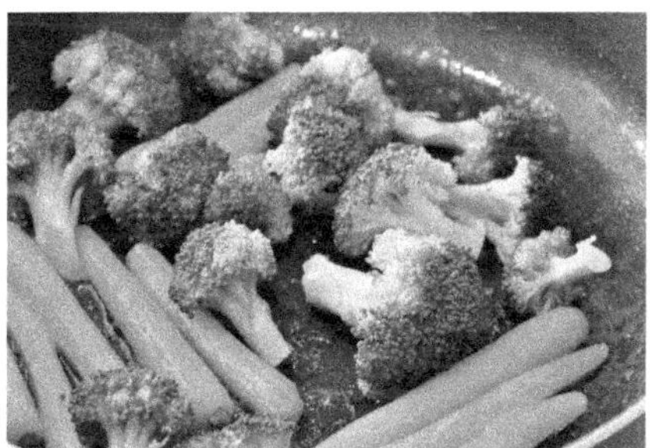

Microwave: Use microwave-safe containers and cover food with a microwave-safe lid or microwave-safe plastic wrap to prevent splatters. Stirring food during reheating helps distribute heat evenly.

Oven: Preheat your oven, and use an oven-safe dish to reheat. Cover with foil to prevent drying out, and use a meat thermometer to ensure safe internal temperatures.

Stovetop: Reheat in a saucepan or skillet over low to medium heat, stirring frequently. Add a bit of liquid (e.g., water or broth) to prevent sticking or drying.

Safe Temperatures: Reheat leftovers to a safe internal temperature of at least 165°F (74°C) to kill bacteria.

Always use common sense and judgment when reheating food. Some foods may not reheat well or may lose quality when reheated multiple times. Additionally, when in doubt about the safety of stored or reheated food, it's better to discard it to avoid foodborne illnesses.

List of equipment used in plant-based diet

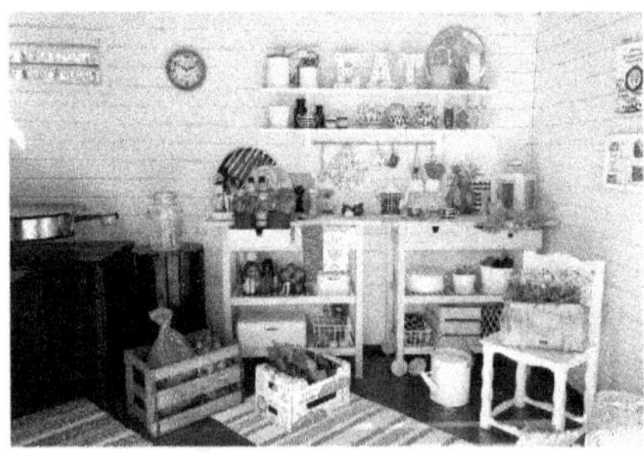

A plant-based diet primarily relies on foods derived from plants, such as fruits, vegetables, grains, nuts, seeds, and legumes. While you don't need specialized equipment to follow a plant-based diet, some kitchen tools can make it easier to prepare and enjoy plant-based meals. Here's a list of equipment commonly used in a plant-based diet:

Blender: Useful for making smoothies, soups, and sauces from fruits and vegetables.

Food Processor: Great for chopping, slicing, and shredding vegetables, as well as making nut-based spreads and energy balls.

High-Speed Blender: Ideal for blending tough ingredients like frozen fruits and nuts into creamy textures.

Juicer: If you enjoy fresh fruit and vegetable juices.

Mandoline Slicer: Helpful for precision slicing of vegetables and fruits.

Salad Spinner: Makes it easy to clean and dry leafy greens and herbs.

Steamer Basket: Useful for steaming vegetables while retaining their nutrients.

Rice Cooker: Perfect for cooking various grains like rice, quinoa, and millet.

Instant Pot or Pressure Cooker: Versatile for cooking beans, lentils, grains, and stews quickly.

Non-Stick Cookware: Useful for sautéing vegetables with minimal oil.

Baking Sheets and Pans: For roasting vegetables, making baked goods, or cooking oil-free fries.

Vegetable Spiralizer: Creates vegetable "noodles" from zucchini, sweet potatoes, and more.

Nut Milk Bag: Essential for making homemade nut or plant-based milk.

Tofu Press: Helps remove excess moisture from tofu, making it firmer and easier to cook with.

Grill or Grill Pan: Great for grilling vegetables and plant-based burgers.

Slow Cooker: Convenient for simmering soups, stews, and beans.

Large Salad Bowl: For tossing together big plant-based salads.

Measuring Cups and Spoons: For accurate ingredient measurements in recipes.

Kitchen Knife Set: Quality knives for chopping, slicing, and dicing vegetables.

Cutting Boards: A variety of cutting boards for different ingredients to avoid cross-contamination.

Food Storage Containers: To store leftovers and meal prep.

While you don't need all of these items to follow a plant-based diet, having some of them can make meal preparation and cooking more efficient and enjoyable. Choose the equipment that suits your cooking style and the types of plant-based dishes you like to prepare.

CHAPTER FOUR

Foods to eat and those to avoid while on a plant-based diet

A plant-based diet is centered around foods derived from plants and excludes or minimizes animal products. Here's a comprehensive list of permitted and non-permitted foods for someone following a plant-based diet:

Permitted Foods (Plant-Based)

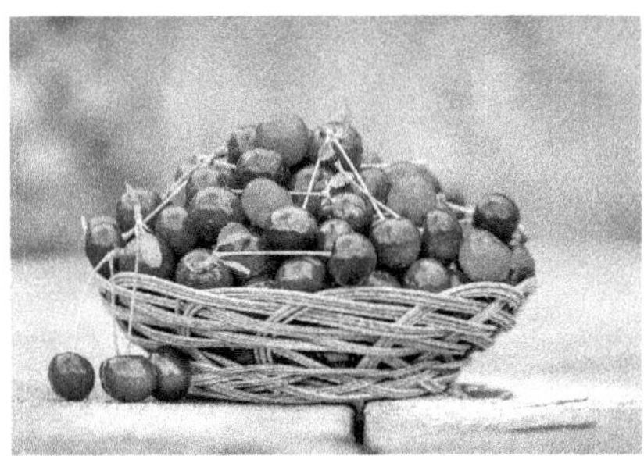

Fruits: All types of fruits, such as apples, bananas, berries, citrus, and more.

Vegetables: A wide variety of vegetables, including leafy greens, root vegetables, cruciferous vegetables, and more.

Grains: Whole grains like rice, quinoa, oats, barley, and whole wheat.

Legumes: Beans, lentils, chickpeas, and peas are excellent sources of plant-based protein.

Nuts: Almonds, walnuts, cashews, and others provide healthy fats and protein.

Seeds: Chia seeds, flaxseeds, sunflower seeds, and pumpkin seeds are common choices.

Plant-Based Milk: Soy milk, almond milk, oat milk, and more as dairy alternatives.

Plant-Based Yogurt: produced from soy, almond, or coconut milk.

Tofu and Tempeh: Versatile sources of plant-based protein.

Herbs and Spices: Enhance flavors without animal products.

Plant Oils: Olive oil, coconut oil, and others for cooking.

Whole Plant-Based Foods: Unprocessed foods are encouraged for maximum health benefits.

Plant-Based Protein Sources: Including seitan (wheat gluten) and plant-based protein powders.

Whole-grain pasta and Bread: Made from whole wheat, rice, or other plant-based flour.

Plant-Based Condiments: Mustard, ketchup, hot sauce, and more.

Plant-Based Sweeteners: Maple syrup, agave nectar, and others in moderation.

Non-Permitted Foods (Generally Excluded on a Plant-Based Diet):

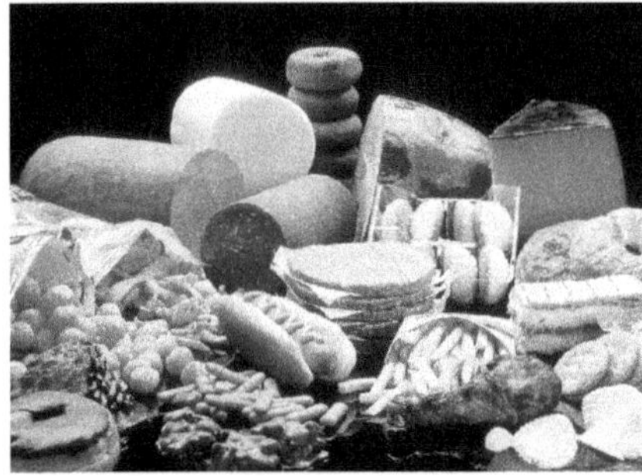

Animal Products: This includes meat, flesh, fish, and seafood.

Dairy Products: Milk, cheese, yogurt, and butter from animal sources.

Eggs: Eggs are from animals and are not considered plant-based.

Honey: Some plant-based eaters avoid honey due to its bee-derived nature.

Gelatin: A product derived from animal collagen.

Processed Foods with Animal Ingredients: Some processed foods contain hidden animal-derived ingredients like gelatin, rennet, or certain food colorings.

It's important to note that there are variations within the plant-based diet. Some people may choose to include occasional animal products or animal-derived ingredients, while others adhere strictly to a vegan or fully plant-based diet. The specific foods consumed can vary based on individual preferences and ethical considerations.

Always read food labels carefully when following a plant-based diet to ensure that products do not contain hidden animal-derived ingredients. Additionally, consulting with a healthcare provider or registered dietitian can be helpful to ensure you're meeting your nutritional needs on a plant-based diet.

Shopping list for someone on a plant grounded diet

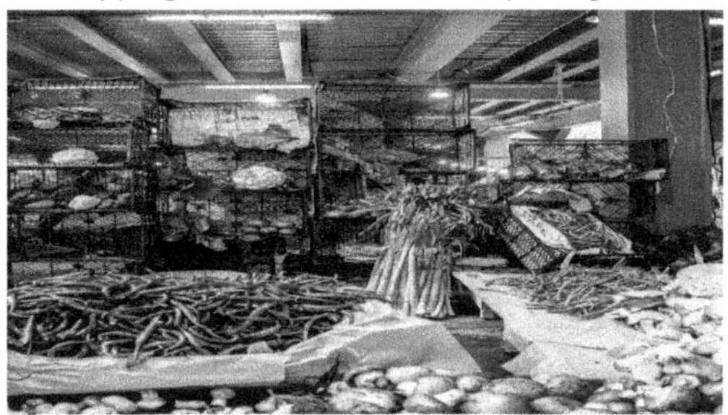

Creating a shopping list for someone on a plant-based diet involves selecting a variety of plant-based foods to ensure a balanced and nutritious diet. Here's a shopping list that includes essential items for a plant-based diet:

Fruits:

Apples

Bananas

Berries (strawberries, blueberries, raspberries)

Citrus fruits (oranges, lemons, limes)

Avocado

Grapes

Kiwi

Mango

Pineapple

Vegetables:

10. Leafy greens (spinach, kale, lettuce)

Tomatoes

Bell peppers

Carrots

Broccoli

Cauliflower

Zucchini

Cucumbers

Onions

Garlic

Legumes:

20. Chickpeas

Black beans

Lentils (green, brown, or red)

Kidney beans

Pinto beans

Grains:

25. Brown rice

Quinoa

Whole wheat pasta

Oats (for oatmeal or baking)

Whole wheat bread

Nuts and Seeds:

30. Almonds

Walnuts

Chia seeds

Flaxseeds

Sunflower seeds

Plant-Based Protein Sources:

35. Tofu

Tempeh

Seitan

Plant-based protein powder (optional)

Plant-Based Dairy Alternatives:

39. Almond milk

Soy milk

Oat milk

Plant-based yogurt (soy, almond, coconut)

Fats and Oils:

43. Olive oil

Coconut oil (for cooking or baking)

Avocado oil (for high-heat cooking)

Nut butter (peanut, almond, or cashew)

Herbs and Spices:

47. Basil

Oregano

Cumin

Paprika

Turmeric

Cinnamon

Garlic powder

Onion powder

Condiments and Sauces:

55. Soy sauce or tamari (for stir-frying)

Tahini

Balsamic vinegar

Hot sauce

Mustard

Plant-based salad dressings

Whole-Plant Foods:

61. Whole-grain cereal

Dried fruits (raisins, apricots)

Canned or dried beans and lentils (for convenience)

Frozen Foods:

64. Frozen fruits (for smoothies)

Frozen vegetables (for quick meals)

Plant-Based Snacks:

66. Popcorn kernels (for air-popping)

Rice cakes

Hummus

Veggie chips

Plant-Based Sweeteners:

70. Maple syrup

Agave nectar

Date syrup

Flashback that this list is just a starting point. Depending on your specific dietary preferences and meal plans, you may need to customize your shopping list. It's also a good idea to include any specialty items or ingredients for specific recipes you plan to make during the week. Lastly, always check labels to ensure products are truly plant-based and free from animal-derived ingredients.

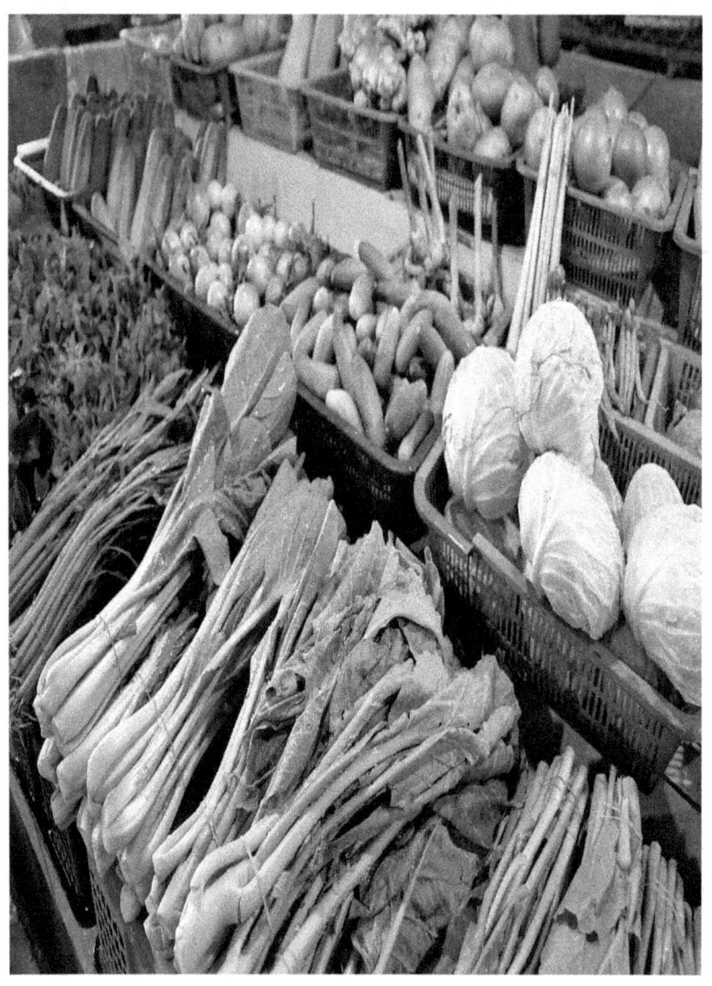

CHAPTER FIVE

Daily Meal Plan and Recipes

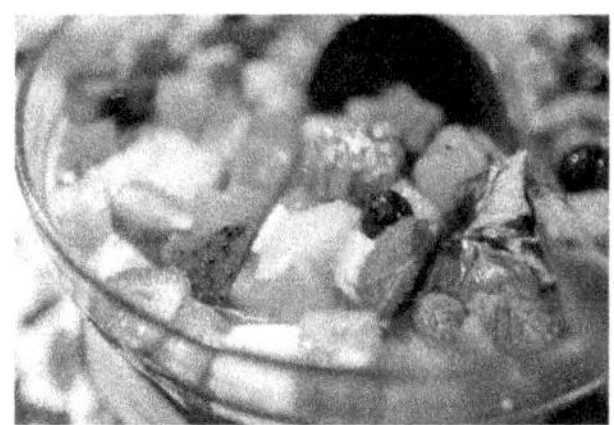

Here are some plant-based breakfast ideas to kickstart your day.

Oatmeal: Cook rolled oats with almond milk or water and top with sliced bananas, berries, nuts, and a drizzle of maple syrup.

Smoothie: Blend frozen fruits (e.g., berries, mango), a banana, spinach, or kale, plant-based yogurt, and a scoop of chia seeds or plant-based protein powder.

Avocado Toast: Spread mashed avocado on whole-grain toast and sprinkle with salt, pepper, and red pepper flakes. Add sliced tomatoes or radishes for extra flavor.

Chia Pudding: Mix chia seeds with almond milk and a touch of sweetener (like maple syrup). Let it sit in the fridge overnight and top it with berries or sliced fruit in the morning.

Pancakes: Make fluffy pancakes using plant-based milk (e.g., almond or oat) and substitute eggs with flaxseed or chia seed "eggs."

Tofu Scramble: Sauté crumbled tofu with onions, bell peppers, spinach, and your favorite spices for a savory breakfast.

Granola and Yogurt: Enjoy plant-based yogurt (e.g., almond or soy) topped with granola, nuts, seeds, and a drizzle of agave syrup.

Fruit Salad: Combine a variety of fresh fruits like melons, berries, and citrus. Squeeze fresh lime or lemon juice for extra zing.

Peanut Butter Banana Sandwich: Spread peanut or almond butter on whole-grain bread and add sliced bananas for a quick and satisfying breakfast.

Breakfast Burrito: Fill a whole-grain tortilla with black beans, sautéed veggies, avocado, and salsa.

Muesli: Combine rolled oats, nuts, seeds, dried fruits, and plant-based yogurt. Let it sit in the fridge overnight for a no-cook breakfast.

Vegan Waffles: Make waffles using plant-based milk and flaxseed or chia seed "eggs." Top with fruit and a drizzle of syrup.

Rice Cakes with Nut Butter: Spread almond or cashew butter on rice cakes and top with sliced strawberries or figs.

Savory Breakfast Bowl: Mix cooked quinoa or brown rice with sautéed greens, roasted sweet potatoes, and a tahini dressing.

Energy Bars: Prepare homemade energy bars with oats, nuts, dried fruits, and a binding agent like dates or nut butter.

Feel free to customize these breakfast ideas to suit your taste and dietary preferences. Plant-based breakfasts can be nutritious, delicious, and versatile.

LUNCH AND DINNER RECIPES:

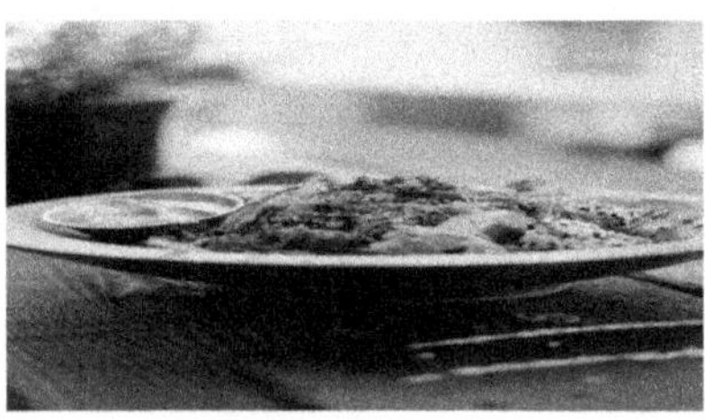

Here are some delicious and nutritious plant-based lunch and dinner recipes:

1. Chickpea and Vegetable Stir-Fry: Ingredients: Chickpeas, broccoli, bell peppers, carrots, snap peas, garlic, ginger, soy sauce, and sesame oil.

Method: Sauté vegetables and chickpeas in a wok with garlic, ginger, and sauce until tender. Serve over brown rice or quinoa.

2. Vegan Lentil Soup:

Ingredients: Green or brown lentils, onion, carrots, celery, garlic, vegetable broth, tomatoes, and spices.

Method: Cook lentils and vegetables in broth with spices until tender for a comforting soup.

3. Vegan Tofu and Vegetable Curry:

Ingredients: Tofu, mixed vegetables, coconut milk, curry paste, garlic, and ginger.

Method: Sauté tofu and vegetables, then simmer in a flavorful curry sauce. Serve with rice or naan bread.

4. Vegan Mushroom Risotto:

Ingredients: Arborio rice, mushrooms, vegetable broth, onion, garlic, white wine, nutritional yeast, and thyme.

Method: Sauté mushrooms and onions, then cook the rice in broth and wine. Stir in nutritive yeast for a ticky-tacky flavor.

5. Vegan Quinoa Salad:

Ingredients: Cooked quinoa, cherry tomatoes, cucumber, red onion, olives, fresh herbs, lemon juice, and olive oil.

Method: Toss all ingredients together for a refreshing salad.

6. Vegan Black Bean Burrito Bowl:

Ingredients: Black beans, cooked rice, corn, avocado, salsa, lime, and cilantro.

Method: Assemble ingredients in a bowl and drizzle with lime juice and salsa.

7. Vegan Spaghetti Aglio e Olio:

Ingredients: Whole wheat spaghetti, garlic, red pepper flakes, olive oil, parsley, and lemon zest.

Method: Sauté garlic and red pepper flakes in olive oil, toss with cooked pasta and garnish with parsley and lemon zest.

8. Vegan Sweet Potato and Chickpea Curry:

Ingredients: Sweet potatoes, chickpeas, coconut milk, curry spices, onion, garlic, and spinach.

Method: Simmer sweet potatoes and chickpeas in a coconut curry sauce, adding spinach at the end.

9. Vegan Veggie Burger:

Ingredients: Chickpeas or black beans, oats, vegetables, spices, and your choice of burger toppings.

Method: Blend ingredients, form into patties, and bake or grill. Serve on a whole wheat bun with your favorite dressings.

10. Vegan Mediterranean Bowl:

- Ingredients: Roasted eggplant, cherry tomatoes, cucumber, olives, quinoa, hummus, and tahini dressing.

- Method: Assemble ingredients in a bowl and drizzle with tahini dressing.

These recipes offer a range of flavors and textures, making them suitable for various preferences and occasions. Feel free to adjust ingredients and seasonings to suit your taste, and enjoy your plant-based lunch and dinner options!

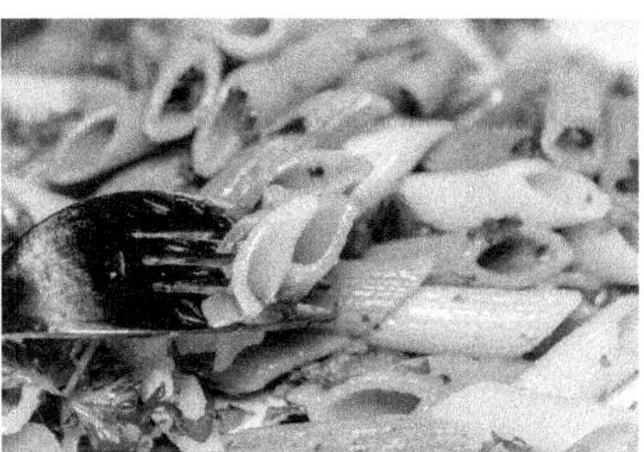

Salads are a fantastic way to incorporate a variety of fresh and healthy ingredients into your meals. Here are some plant-based salad ideas:

Classic Garden Salad:

Ingredients: Lettuce, tomatoes, cucumbers, bell peppers, red onions, and olives.

Dressing: Balsamic vinaigrette or a lemon-tahini dressing.

Greek Salad:

Ingredients: Cucumbers, cherry tomatoes, red onions, kalamata olives, and vegan feta cheese (made from tofu or almonds).

Dressing: Olive oil, lemon juice, garlic, and oregano.

Caesar Salad:

Ingredients: Romaine lettuce, croutons (make them from whole-grain bread), and vegan Caesar dressing.

Optional: Vegan parmesan cheese or nutritional yeast.

Quinoa Salad:

Ingredients: Cooked quinoa, diced bell peppers, cherry tomatoes, cucumber, red onion, and fresh herbs (parsley or cilantro).

Dressing: Lemon vinaigrette or a tahini-based dressing.

Mediterranean Chickpea Salad:

Ingredients: Chickpeas, cherry tomatoes, cucumber, red onion, olives, and fresh parsley.

Dressing: Olive oil, lemon juice, garlic, and dried oregano.

Asian-Inspired Salad:

Ingredients: Shredded cabbage, carrots, bell peppers, edamame, and sliced almonds.

Dressing: Sesame ginger dressing or peanut sauce.

Kale and Avocado Salad:

Ingredients: Massaged kale, avocado slices, cherry tomatoes, and pine nuts.

Dressing: Lemon-tahini dressing.

Roasted Vegetable Salad:

Ingredients: Roasted sweet potatoes, beets, carrots, and red onion on a bed of mixed greens.

Dressing: Balsamic vinaigrette.

Fruit Salad with Greens:

Ingredients: Mixed greens, sliced strawberries, blueberries, and candied pecans.

Dressing: A light raspberry vinaigrette.

Bean Salad:

Ingredients: A mix of canned or cooked beans (like kidney beans, black beans, and chickpeas), diced bell peppers, red onion, and corn.

Dressing: Lime-cilantro vinaigrette.

Tofu Salad:

Ingredients: Marinated and baked tofu cubes, mixed greens, cherry tomatoes, cucumber, and sliced radishes.

Dressing: Sesame ginger or miso dressing.

Panzanella Salad:

Ingredients: Cubed whole-grain bread, cherry tomatoes, cucumber, red onion, and fresh basil.

Dressing: Olive oil, balsamic vinegar, and garlic.

Remember to get creative with your salads by adding your favorite toppings, nuts, seeds, and protein sources like beans or tofu. Also, consider making your dressings using olive oil, vinegar, lemon juice, and herbs for a healthier and more flavorful option. Enjoy your plant-based salads!

Bowl

Bowls have become a popular way to enjoy a balanced and visually appealing meal, often featuring a variety of ingredients layered together. Here are some plant-based bowl ideas you can try:

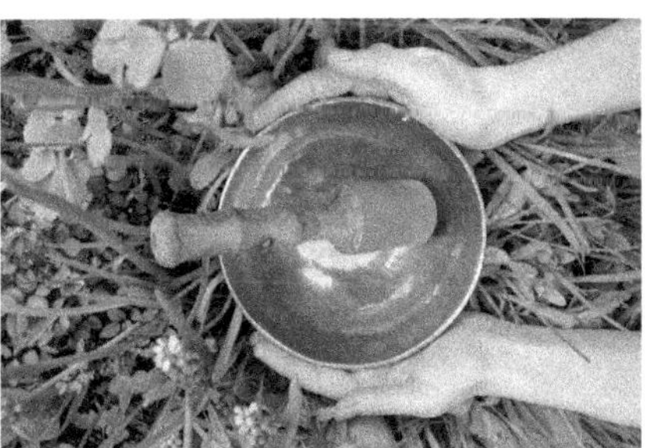

Buddha Bowl:

Base: Quinoa or brown rice.

Protein: Baked tofu or chickpeas.

Vegetables: Steamed or roasted broccoli, carrots, and bell peppers.

Greens: Baby spinach or kale.

Toppings: Avocado slices, sesame seeds, and a tahini dressing.

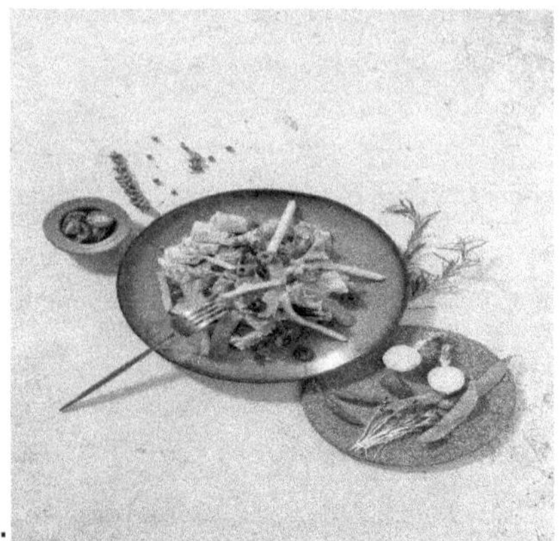

Burrito Bowl:

Base: Brown rice or cauliflower rice.

Protein: Black beans or lentils cooked with Mexican spices.

Vegetables: Sautéed bell peppers, onions, and corn.

Toppings: Salsa, guacamole, diced tomatoes, and fresh cilantro.

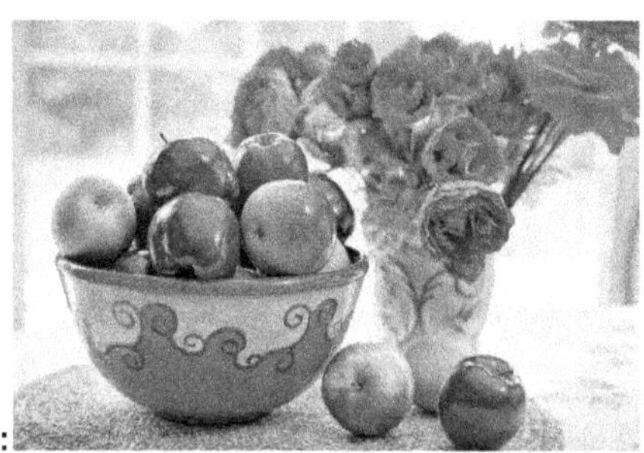

Mediterranean Bowl:

Base: Quinoa or couscous.

Protein: Falafel or grilled tempeh.

Vegetables: Cucumber, cherry tomatoes, red onion, and kalamata olives.

Greens: Romaine lettuce or arugula.

Toppings: Hummus and a lemon-tahini dressing.

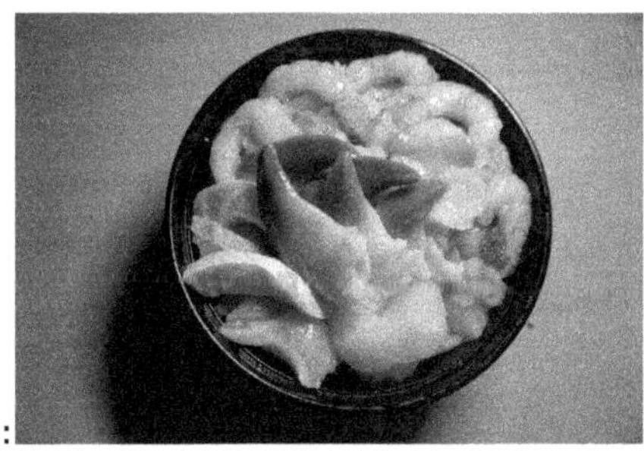

Sushi Bowl:

Base: Sushi rice or brown rice.

Protein: Marinated tofu or edamame.

Vegetables: Sliced cucumber, avocado, and shredded carrots.

Toppings: Pickled ginger, nori seaweed strips, and soy sauce or tamari.

Poke Bowl:

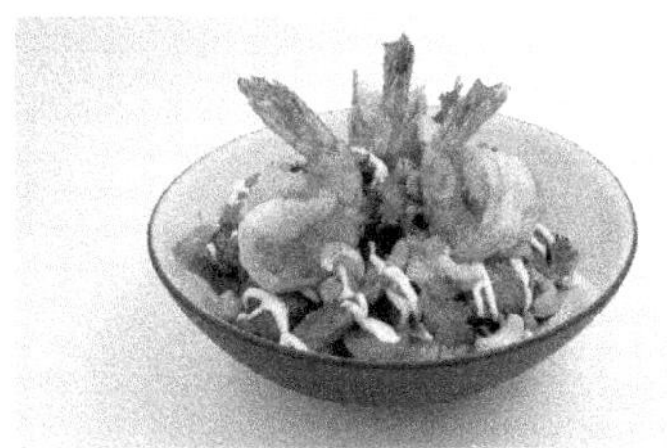

Base: Sushi rice or brown rice.

Protein: Marinated tofu or diced tempeh.

Vegetables: Sliced cucumber, edamame, and seaweed salad.

Toppings: Sesame seeds, sliced avocado, and a spicy mayo or soy-sesame dressing.

Mexican Quinoa Bowl:

Base: Quinoa.

Protein: Black beans or pinto beans.

Vegetables: Roasted sweet potatoes, corn, and red onion.

Toppings: Salsa, guacamole, and fresh cilantro.

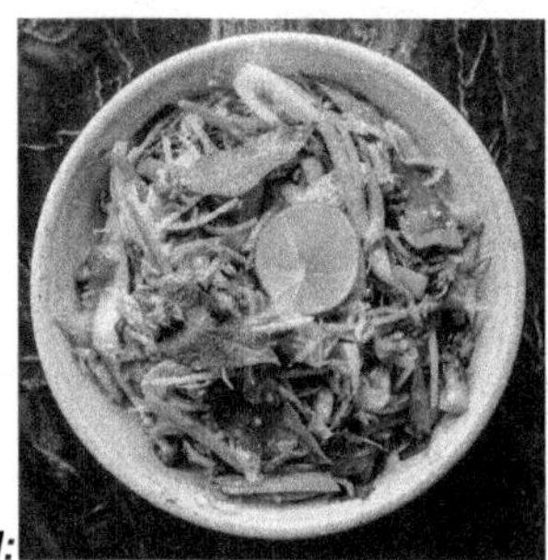

Thai Noodle Bowl:

Base: Rice noodles or zucchini noodles.

Protein: Tofu or tempeh.

Vegetables: Sautéed or steamed broccoli, bell peppers, and snap peas.

Toppings: Chopped peanuts, fresh lime, and a peanut sauce.

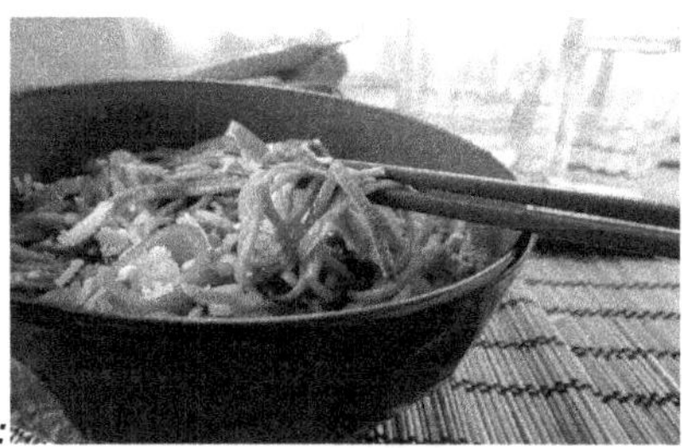

Soba Noodle Bowl:

Base: Soba noodles.

Protein: Baked tofu or edamame.

Vegetables: Sliced cucumber, shredded carrots, and steamed bok choy.

Toppings: Green onions, sesame seeds, and a soy-ginger dressing.

These are just a many ideas to get you started. Feel free to mix and match ingredients, sauces, and toppings to create your own delicious and nutritious plant-based bowls. The key is to balance flavors, textures, and colors for a satisfying meal.

Stews and soups recipes

Stews and soups are versatile and comforting dishes that can easily be made plant-based. Here are some plant-based stew and soup ideas:

Stews

Vegetable Stew:

Ingredients: Potatoes, carrots, celery, peas, corn, and green beans.

Flavor: Simmer in a vegetable broth with herbs like thyme and rosemary.

Chickpea and Spinach Stew:

Ingredients: Chickpeas, spinach, tomatoes, and onions.

Flavor: Add spices like cumin, coriander, and paprika for depth.

Lentil Stew:

Ingredients: Brown or green lentils, carrots, onions, and celery.

Flavor: Use vegetable broth and season with bay leaves and garlic.

Vegan Chili: Ingredients: Kidney beans, black beans, tomatoes, bell peppers, and onions.

Flavor: Chili powder, cumin, and smoked paprika for a smoky kick.

Sweet Potato and Black Bean Stew:

Ingredients: Sweet potatoes, black beans, tomatoes, and corn.

Flavor: Add chipotle peppers in adobo sauce for a spicy, smoky flavor.

Soups

Minestrone Soup:

Ingredients: Pasta, white beans, tomatoes, carrots, zucchini, and spinach.

Flavor: Season with Italian herbs like basil and oregano.

Tomato Basil Soup:

Ingredients: Tomatoes, onions, garlic, and fresh basil.

Flavor: Blend until smooth and finish with a drizzle of olive oil.

Curried Coconut Lentil Soup:

Ingredients: Red lentils, coconut milk, carrots, and curry spices.

Flavor: Create a fragrant broth with curry powder, turmeric, and ginger.

Vegan Potato Leek Soup:

Ingredients: Potatoes, leeks, onions, and garlic.

Flavor: Simmer with vegetable broth and garnish with fresh chives.

Mushroom Barley Soup:

Ingredients: Mushrooms, barley, carrots, celery, and onions.

Flavor: Enhance with thyme and a splash of soy sauce.

Spicy Thai Noodle Soup:

Ingredients: Rice noodles, tofu or tempeh, mushrooms, and bok choy.

Flavor: Create a spicy, tangy broth with lemongrass, ginger, and red curry paste.

Remember to adjust the seasoning and spices to suit your taste preferences, and don't be afraid to experiment with different vegetables and legumes in your stews and soups. Serve with a side of crusty bread or a green salad for a complete and satisfying meal.

Pastas and grains recipes

Certainly! Pasta and grains are versatile staples in a plant-based diet. Here are some plant-based pasta and grain dish ideas:

Pasta

Classic Spaghetti Marinara:

Ingredients: Whole wheat or gluten-free spaghetti with tomato sauce (with garlic, onions, basil, and oregano).

Topping: Sprinkle with nutritional yeast or vegan parmesan.

Pesto Pasta:

Ingredients: Pasta of your choice with homemade or store-bought basil pesto (blend basil, garlic, nuts, and olive oil).

Add: Cherry tomatoes, roasted pine nuts, and vegan parmesan.

Vegan Alfredo Pasta:

Ingredients: Fettuccine or linguine with a creamy cashew-based Alfredo sauce.

Add: Sautéed mushrooms, peas, and spinach.

Lemon Garlic Pasta:

Ingredients: Linguine or spaghetti with a lemony garlic sauce.

Add: Sautéed asparagus or broccoli and sprinkle with fresh parsley.

Vegan Mac and Cheese:

Ingredients: Elbow macaroni with a creamy sauce made from cashews, nutritional yeast, and plant-based milk.

Optional: Top with breadcrumbs and bake for a crispy crust.

Grains

Quinoa Salad:

Ingredients: Cooked quinoa mixed with diced cucumbers, tomatoes, red onions, and fresh herbs.

Dressing: Lemon vinaigrette or a tahini-based dressing.

Vegan Fried Rice:

Ingredients: Cooked brown rice with sautéed tofu or tempeh, mixed vegetables, and soy sauce.

Flavor: Add garlic, ginger, and sesame oil for extra taste.

Veggie Stir-Fry with Rice:

Ingredients: Brown rice with a stir-fry of broccoli, bell peppers, carrots, and snap peas.

Sauce: Make a savory stir-fry sauce using soy sauce or tamari, garlic, and ginger.

Couscous and Chickpea Salad:

Ingredients: Cooked couscous mixed with chickpeas, diced cucumbers, cherry tomatoes, and fresh mint.

Dressing: Lemon and olive oil dressing with a touch of cumin.

Vegan Risotto:

Ingredients: Arborio rice cooked with vegetable broth, mushrooms, and onions.

Finish with: Nutritional yeast or vegan parmesan and fresh parsley.

Barley and Vegetable Soup:

Ingredients: Cooked barley with a hearty vegetable broth, carrots, celery, and peas.

Flavor: Add thyme and rosemary for depth.

Remember to choose whole grains for added nutrition and fiber in your pasta and grain dishes. You can customize these dishes with your favorite vegetables and seasonings to suit your taste preferences. Plant-based eating can be delicious and nutritious with a variety of pasta and grain-based meals.

Appetizers and Snacks

Plant-based appetizers and snacks can be both delicious and satisfying. Here are some ideas for plant-based appetizers and snacks:

Appetizers:

Guacamole and Salsa: Serve with tortilla chips or veggie sticks.

Hummus Platter: Offer a variety of hummus flavors with pita bread, cucumber, carrot, and bell pepper sticks.

Stuffed Mushrooms: Fill mushroom caps with a mixture of breadcrumbs, garlic, herbs, and vegan cream cheese.

Vegan Spring Rolls: Rice paper rolls filled with rice noodles, tofu, herbs, and veggies, served with peanut sauce.

Vegan Bruschetta: Top toasted baguette slices with diced tomatoes, garlic, basil, and a drizzle of balsamic vinegar.

Cauliflower Buffalo Wings: Coat cauliflower flowerets in a spicy buffalo sauce and singe until crisp.

Vegan Spinach and Artichoke Dip: Make a creamy dip using cashews and nutritional yeast, then mix in spinach and artichoke hearts.

Vegan Sushi Rolls: Roll sushi with avocado, cucumber, carrots, and marinated tofu, served with soy sauce and wasabi.

Vegan Quesadillas: Fill tortillas with vegan cheese, black beans, corn, and bell peppers, then cook until crispy.

Vegan Caprese Skewers: Thread cherry tomatoes, basil leaves, and vegan mozzarella onto skewers, and drizzle with balsamic glaze.

Snacks:

Trail Mix: Combine nuts, seeds, dried fruits, and a touch of dark chocolate.

Popcorn: Air-pop popcorn and season with nutritional yeast or your favorite seasoning.

Fruit Salad: Chop a variety of fresh fruits and drizzle with lime juice and a sprinkle of chili powder.

Veggie Sticks and Dip: Serve carrot, celery, cucumber, and bell pepper sticks with hummus or a vegan ranch dip.

Rice Cakes with Nut Butter: Spread almond or peanut butter on rice cakes and top with sliced banana.

Energy Balls: Blend dates, nuts, seeds, and a touch of cocoa powder, then roll into bite-sized balls.

Frozen Grapes: A refreshing and naturally sweet snack straight from the freezers.

Chia Pudding: Make chia seed pudding with almond milk and top with pristine berries.

Roasted Chickpeas: Toss chickpeas with olive oil and spices, then roast until crunchy.

Vegan Yogurt Parfait: Layer plant-based yogurt with granola and mixed berries in a glass.

These appetizers and snacks are not only plant-based but also packed with flavor and nutrition. Whether you're serving them at a gathering or enjoying them as a quick bite, there are plenty of delicious options to choose from.

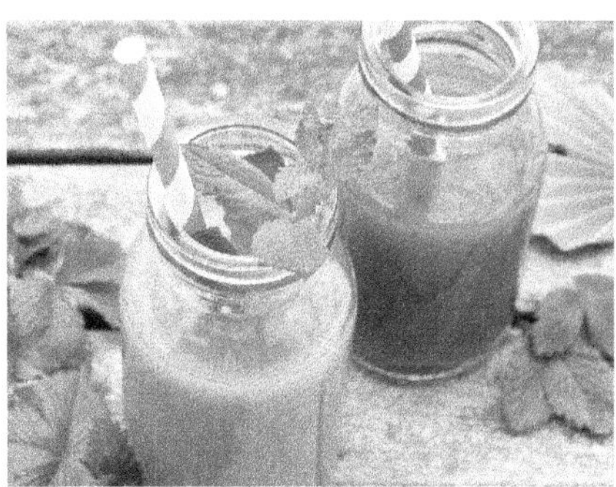

Smoothies Recipes

Certainly! Here are some delicious plant-based smoothie recipes for you to try:

1. Berry Blast Smoothie:

1 cup mixed berries (strawberries, blueberries, raspberries)

1 banana

1 cup spinach or kale leaves

1 tablespoon chia seeds

1 mug almond milk(or your preferred plant-based milk)

Optional sweetener: 1-2 teaspoons of maple syrup or agave nectar

2. Green Tropical Smoothie:

1 cup pineapple chunks (fresh or frozen)

1/2 banana

1 cup spinach or kale leaves

1/2 cup coconut milk

1/2 cup orange juice

Optional: 1 tablespoon shredded coconut

3. Peanut Butter Banana Smoothie:

2 ripe bananas

2 tablespoons peanut butter (or almond butter)

1 cup plant-based yogurt

1 cup almond milk

1 tablespoon flaxseed meal

Optional a sprinkle of maple syrup for a pleasant taste

4. Chocolate Avocado Smoothie:

1 ripe avocado

2 tablespoons cocoa powder

1 banana

1 cup almond milk.

1 teaspoon agave beverage(or sweetener of your choice)

A pinch of salt

5. Mango Madness Smoothie:

1 1/2 cups frozen mango chunks

1/2 banana

1 cup coconut water

1/2 cup orange juice

1 tablespoon chia seeds

6. Oatmeal Cookie Smoothie:

1/2 cup rolled oats

1 banana

1/2 teaspoon ground cinnamon

1 tablespoon almond butter

1 cup almond milk

A dash of vanilla extract

7. Blueberry Almond Bliss Smoothie:

1 cup blueberries (fresh or frozen)

2 tablespoons almond butter

1 cup spinach leaves

1 tablespoon flaxseed meal

1 cup almond milk

8. Pineapple Ginger Zinger:

1 cup pineapple chunks (fresh or frozen)

1-inch piece of fresh ginger

1/2 banana

1 cup coconut water

A squeeze of lime juice

9. Very Berry Protein Smoothie:

1/2 cup mixed berries (strawberries, blueberries, raspberries)

1/2 cup silken tofu or plant-based protein powder

1 banana

1 cup almond milk

1 tablespoon honey or maple syrup to taste

10. Chai Spice Smoothie:

- 1 banana

- 1/2 teaspoon ground cinnamon

- 1/4 teaspoon ground cardamom

- 1/4 teaspoon ground ginger

- 1/4 teaspoon ground cloves

- 1/4 teaspoon ground nutmeg

- 1 cup chai-spiced plant-based milk (or regular plant-based milk)

Feel free to adjust the sweetness, thickness, or consistency of these smoothies to your liking. You can also add ice cubes for a colder version or adjust the quantity of liquid for a thicker or thinner texture. Enjoy your plant-based smoothies!

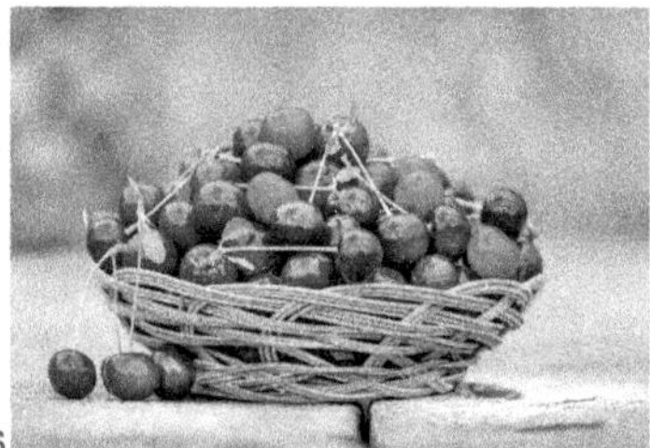

Desserts

Plant-based desserts can be just as indulgent and delicious as traditional desserts. Here are some mouthwatering plant-based dessert ideas:

1. Vegan Chocolate Avocado Mousse:

Ingredients: Ripe avocados, cocoa powder, maple syrup, and vanilla extract.

Method: Blend until smooth, chill, and serve with berries or nuts.

2. Vegan Banana Ice Cream:

Ingredients: Frozen ripe bananas.

Method: Blend frozen bananas until creamy. Add Seasonings like vanilla extract or cocoa powder.

3. Vegan Chocolate Chip Cookies:

Ingredients: Flour, dairy-free chocolate chips, coconut oil, and sugar.

Method: Mix, bake, and enjoy warm, gooey cookies.

4. Vegan Berry Parfait:

Ingredients: Layers of plant-based yogurt, mixed berries, and granola.

Method: Assemble in a glass, repeat layers, and drizzle with agave nectar.

5. Vegan Rice Pudding:

Ingredients: Rice, almond milk, sugar, and cinnamon.

Method: Simmer rice in almond milk, sweeten, and season with cinnamon.

6. Vegan Chocolate Fondue:

Ingredients: Melted dairy-free chocolate with coconut milk.

Serve with strawberries, banana slices, or marshmallows for dipping.

7. Vegan Apple Crisp:

Ingredients: Sliced apples, oats, almond meal, maple syrup, and cinnamon.

Method: Mix and bake until the topping is golden and crispy.

8. Vegan Chia Seed Pudding:

Ingredients: Chia seeds, almond milk, and sweetener (maple syrup, agave).

Method: Mix and refrigerate overnight. Top with fruit and nuts.

9. Vegan Peanut Butter Cups:

Ingredients: Dairy-free chocolate chips, peanut butter, and a touch of sweetener.

Method: Melt chocolate, fill molds with peanut butter mixture, and chill.

10. Vegan Coconut Bliss Balls:

- Ingredients: Dates, shredded coconut, nuts, and cocoa powder.

- Method: Blend, roll into balls, and coat with extra coconut or cocoa.

11. Vegan Pumpkin Pie:

- Ingredients: Pumpkin puree, coconut milk, spices, and a vegan pie crust.

- Method: Mix and bake until set.

12. Vegan Cheesecake:

- Ingredients: Cashews, coconut cream, sweetener, and fruit (e.g., strawberries or blueberries).

- Method: Blend filling ingredients, pour into a crust, and chill.

13. Vegan Chocolate Pudding:

- Ingredients: Silken tofu, cocoa powder, maple syrup, and vanilla extract.

- Method: Blend until creamy and refrigerate.

14. Vegan Lemon Bars:

- Ingredients: Almond flour crust and a lemony filling made with lemon juice, zest, and sweetener.

- Method: Bake and cool before slicing.

These plant-based dessert options offer a wide range of flavors and textures to satisfy your sweet tooth while adhering to a plant-based diet. You can adapt and customize these recipes to your preferred tastes and dietary needs.

Plant-based dressings and sauces can add flavor and zest to your meals. Here are some delicious plant-based dressing and sauce recipes:

1. Balsamic Vinaigrette:

Ingredients: Balsamic vinegar, olive oil, Dijon mustard, maple syrup, minced garlic, salt, and pepper.

Method: Whisk or shake ingredients in a jar until emulsified.

2. Lemon-Tahini Dressing:

Ingredients: Tahini, lemon juice, water, minced garlic, maple syrup, salt, and pepper.

Method: Whisk together until smooth, adjusting the water for desired consistency.

3. Vegan Ranch Dressing:

Ingredients: Plant-based yogurt, garlic powder, onion powder, dried dill, dried parsley, apple cider vinegar, salt, and pepper.

Method: Mix all ingredients until well combined.

4. Vegan Caesar Dressing:

Ingredients: Cashews, lemon juice, Dijon mustard, garlic, capers, nutritional yeast, water, salt, and pepper.

Method: Blend until creamy and smooth.

5. Vegan Pesto Sauce:

Ingredients: Fresh basil leaves, pine nuts, garlic, nutritional yeast, olive oil, lemon juice, salt, and pepper.

Method: Blend until it reaches your desired consistency.

6. Thai Peanut Sauce:

Ingredients: Peanut butter, soy sauce or tamari, lime juice, maple syrup, garlic, ginger, and red pepper flakes.

Method: Whisk together or blend until smooth.

7. Vegan Tzatziki Sauce:

Ingredients: Plant-based yogurt, cucumber, lemon juice, dill, garlic, salt, and pepper.

Method: Grate cucumber, squeeze out excess moisture, and mix with other ingredients.

8. Vegan BBQ Sauce:

Ingredients: Ketchup, maple syrup, apple cider vinegar, smoked paprika, garlic powder, onion powder, and a dash of hot sauce.

Method: Mix until well combined and adjust sweetness and spiciness to taste.

9. Sweet Chili Sauce:

Ingredients: Agave nectar or maple syrup, rice vinegar, garlic, red pepper flakes, and cornstarch (for thickening).

Method: Simmer ingredients until thickened, stirring constantly.

10. Vegan Teriyaki Sauce:

- Ingredients: Soy sauce or tamari, water, brown sugar or maple syrup, minced garlic, minced ginger, and cornstarch (for thickening).

- Method: Combine and simmer until thickened, stirring constantly.

These plant-based dressings and sauces can be used to enhance salads, drizzle over roasted vegetables, marinated tofu or tempeh, or as a dipping sauce for various dishes. Adjust the seasonings to your taste preferences, and feel free to experiment with ingredients to create your unique flavors.

CHAPTER SIX

12 WEEKS HEALTHY VEGAN

Embarking on a 12-week journey to a healthy vegan lifestyle is a wonderful choice for your health and the environment. Then is a general plan to help you get started:

Weeks 1-2: Education and Transition

Research plant-based nutrition: Learn about essential nutrients and where to find them in a vegan diet.

Begin by eliminating animal products gradually. Replace meat with plant-based protein sources like tofu, tempeh, and legumes.

Explore vegan recipes and cooking techniques.

Weeks 3-4: Balanced Meal Planning

Focus on balanced meals: Incorporate whole grains, a variety of vegetables, legumes, and plant-based protein sources into your meals.

Experiment with new recipes, including hearty salads, stir-fries, and grain bowls.

Weeks 5-6: Snack Smart

Discover plant-based snacks like nuts, seeds, fruit, veggie sticks with hummus, and plant-based yogurt with granola.

Limit processed snacks and choose whole foods for better nutrition.

Weeks 7-8: Explore New Flavors

Experiment with global cuisines that naturally feature plant-based dishes, such as Indian, Thai, and Mediterranean.

Try new herbs and spices to enhance flavor.

Weeks 9-10: Nutrient-Rich Choices

Pay attention to getting essential nutrients like B12, iron, calcium, and omega-3 fatty acids. Take into account fortified foods or supplements as required.

Include dark leafy greens, beans, lentils, and whole grains in your diet for added nutrition.

Weeks 11-12: Sustainability and Long-Term Goals

Reflect on the environmental benefits of your vegan diet.

Consider reducing processed foods and focusing on whole, plant-based ingredients for better health.

Plan meals to make the transition smoother.

Throughout the 12 Weeks: Lifestyle Adjustments

Gradually replace non-vegan personal care products with cruelty-free alternatives.

Educate yourself on vegan fashion choices.

Engage with the vegan community for support and recipe ideas.

Additional Tips:

Stay hydrated and drink plenty of water.

Prioritize whole foods over processed vegan alternatives.

attend to your body's hunger and wholeness cues.

Keep a food diary to track your nutrient intake initially.

Be patient and kind to yourself during this transition.

Remember, everyone's journey to a healthy vegan lifestyle is unique, so tailor this plan to your specific needs and preferences. Consulting a registered dietitian or nutritionist can also provide personalized guidance to ensure you meet your nutritional goals. Enjoy your 12-week journey to a healthier, more sustainable way of eating!

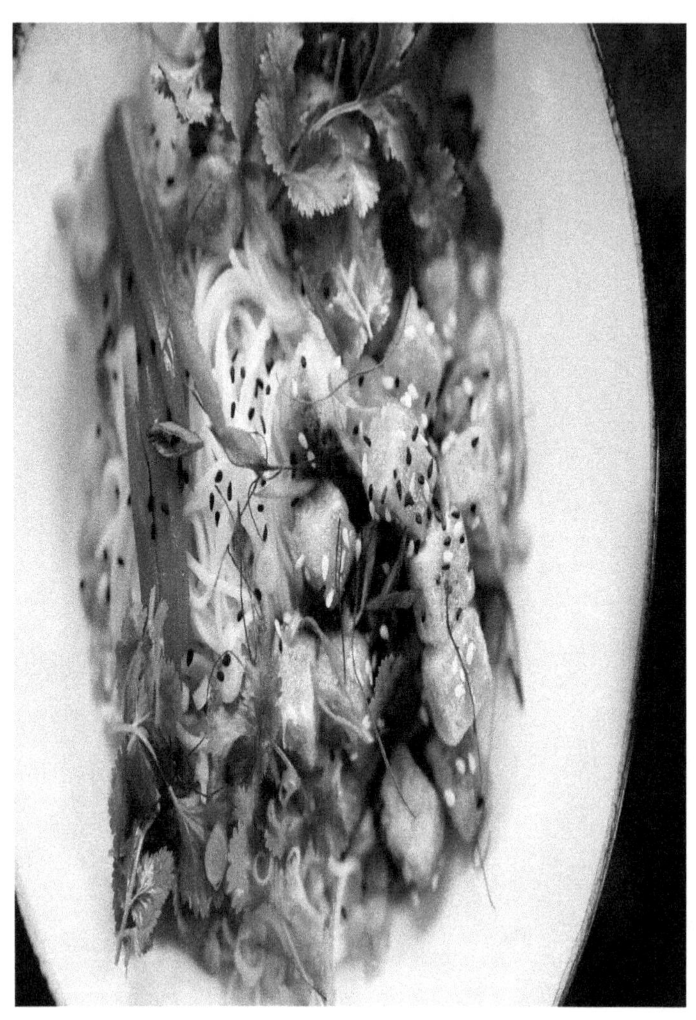

Conclusion

"In conclusion, a plant-based diet offers a myriad of benefits for both different fitness and the surroundings.

Throughout this document, we have explored the various aspects of adopting a plant-based lifestyle, from its definitions and types to its nutritional considerations, health advantages, and sustainability.

By choosing a plant-based diet, individuals can enjoy lower risks of chronic diseases, improved weight management, and enhanced overall well-being. This dietary approach emphasizes the consumption of nutrient-rich foods such as fruits, vegetables, legumes, and whole grains, which are rich sources of essential vitamins, minerals, and antioxidants.

Moreover, the environmental impact of embracing a plant-based diet cannot be understated. It contributes to reduced greenhouse gas emissions, conserves water resources, and helps mitigate deforestation. As our global community becomes increasingly aware of the environmental challenges we face, the transition to plant-based eating stands as a sustainable and impactful choice.

Transitioning to a plant-based diet may present challenges initially, but with the abundance of resources, recipes, and supportive communities available, anyone can embark on this rewarding journey. We encourage individuals to explore the diverse flavors and possibilities that plant-based cuisine offers, experiment with recipes, and reap the numerous health and environmental benefits.

In closing, the adoption of a plant-based diet is not only a personal choice for improved health but also a significant step towards a more sustainable and compassionate future. As more people embrace plant-based eating, we can collectively make a positive impact on our health and the planet. Let us embark on this journey together, mindful of the profound changes it can bring to our lives and our world."

Daily meal remark

Day	Recipes	Remark